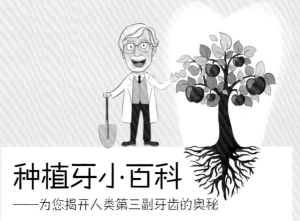

种植牙小·百科
——为您揭开人类第三副牙齿的奥秘

A Small Encyclopedia of Dental Implants
——to discover the mystery of the third dentition

主　编　王少海　马　威
Chief Editors　Shaohai Wang, Wei Ma

副主编　马军萍　孙　健　何　帅
Associate Editors　Junping Bergin, Jian Sun, Shuai He

U0294935

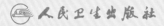

人民卫生出版社

图书在版编目（CIP）数据

种植牙小百科 / 王少海，马威主编 . —北京：人
民卫生出版社，2018

ISBN 978-7-117-27442-5

Ⅰ . ①种… Ⅱ . ①王…②马… Ⅲ . ①种植牙 – 基本
知识 Ⅳ . ①R782.12

中国版本图书馆 CIP 数据核字（2018）第 211169 号

人卫智网	www.ipmph.com	医学教育、学术、考试、健康，
		购书智慧智能综合服务平台
人卫官网	www.pmph.com	人卫官方资讯发布平台

种植牙小百科

主　　编：王少海　马　威
出版发行：人民卫生出版社（中继线 010-59780011）
地　　址：北京市朝阳区潘家园南里 19 号
邮　　编：100021
E - mail：pmph @ pmph.com
购书热线：010-59787592　010-59787584　010-65264830
印　　刷：北京顶佳世纪印刷有限公司
经　　销：新华书店
开　　本：889×1194　1/32　印张：4.5
字　　数：113 千字
版　　次：2018 年 11 月第 1 版　2018 年 11 月第 1 版第 1 次印刷
标准书号：ISBN 978-7-117-27442-5
定　　价：40.00 元

打击盗版举报电话：010-59787491　E-mail：WQ @ pmph.com
（凡属印装质量问题请与本社市场营销中心联系退换）

编者
Contributors
（按姓氏首字母排序）

陈　惠（上海交通大学医学院附属第九人民医院）

陈　彤（海军军医大学附属长海医院）

高建勇（海军军医大学附属长海医院）

何　帅（温州医科大学附属第二医院/育婴儿童医院）

黄争美（上海交通大学医学院附属第九人民医院）

刘　艳（空军军医大学口腔医学院）

马军萍（美国华盛顿大学牙科学院）

马　威（空军军医大学口腔医院）

Luba Pacyga（美国西雅图 Bergin 修复专科诊所）

邱小倩（海军军医大学附属长海医院）

孙　健（上海交通大学医学院附属第九人民医院）

唐　震（海军军医大学附属长海医院）

王宁涛（海军军医大学附属长海医院）

王少海（海军军医大学附属长海医院）

Hsiang Y Yin（美国西雅图 Bergin 修复专科诊所）

祖丽皮也·阿不力克木（海军军医大学附属长海医院）

朱庆丰（海军军医大学附属长海医院）

编者
Contributors

Hui Chen (Shanghai Ninth People's Hospital, Shanghai Jiaotong University, Shanghai, China)

Tong Chen (Changhai Hospital, Navy Military Medical University, Shanghai, China)

Jianyong Gao (Changhai Hospital, Navy Military Medical University, Shanghai, China)

Shuai He (The Second Affiliated Hospital & Yuying Children's Hospital, Wenzhou Medical University, Wenzhou, China)

Zhengmei Huang (Shanghai Ninth People's Hospital, Shanghai Jiaotong University, Shanghai, China)

Yan Liu (School of Stomatology, Air Force Military Medical University, Xi'an, China)

Junping Bergin, D.M.D M.S. (Affiliate faculty, School of Dentistry, University of Washington, Seattle, USA)

Wei Ma (School of Stomatology, Air Force Military Medical University, Xi'an, China)

Luba Pacyga (Bergin Prosthodontics, Seattle, USA)

Xiaoqian Qiu (Changhai Hospital, Navy Military Medical University,

Shanghai, China)

Jian Sun (Shanghai Ninth People's Hospital, Shanghai Jiaotong University, Shanghai, China)

Zhen Tang (Changhai Hospital, Navy Military Medical University, Shanghai, China)

Ningtao Wang (Changhai Hospital, Navy Military Medical University, Shanghai, China)

Shaohai Wang (Changhai Hospital, Navy Military Medical University, Shanghai, China)

Hsiang Y Yin (Bergin Prosthodontics, Seattle, USA)

Zulipiye Ablikim (Changhai Hospital, Navy Military Medical University, Shanghai, China)

Qingfeng Zhu (Changhai Hospital, Navy Military Medical University, Shanghai, China)

主编简介
About the Editors

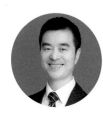

● 王少海博士

海军军医大学(原第二军医大学)附属长海医院口腔科主任医师,教授,研究生导师。现任中华口腔医学会口腔修复专业委员会委员,中华口腔医学会口腔颌面修复专业委员会委员,中国整形美容协会口腔整形美容专业委员会委员,上海市口腔医学会口腔修复学专业委员会委员。主编《口腔种植应用解剖实物图谱》《口腔种植手术学图解》。

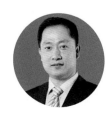

● 马威博士

空军军医大学口腔医学院种植科副主任医师,副教授,研究生导师。现任ICOI(国际口腔种植医师学)中国总会副会长,中华口腔医学会口腔种植专业委员会委员,中国生物材料学会口腔生物材料及应用专业委员会委员,全国卫生产业企业管理协会数字化口腔产业分会专家委员会委员。多次赴欧洲、美国和日本进行学习交流与访问。

● Shaohai Wang, MD

Graduated from Air Force Military Medical University (the Fourth Military Medical University), now working in Navy Military Medical University, Changhai Hospital, Department of Stomatology, professor/chief physician, postgraduate instructor. Council member of prosthetic committee of CSA (Chinese Stomatological Association).Council member of Oral and Maxillofacial rehabilitation committee of CSA (Chinese Stomatological Association).

● Wei Ma, MD

Graduated from Air Force Military Medical University (the Fourth Military Medical University), now working in Air Force Military Medical University School of Stomatology, Department of Dental Implants. Associate professor/associate chief physician, postgraduate instructor. Vice president of Chinese society of ICOI (International Congress of Oral Implantologists), Council member of CSOI (Chinese Society of Oral Implants).

前言
Foreword

　　种植牙是一项成熟的医疗技术，其独有的优势不可比拟。由于技术复杂，科技含量高，患者对该技术多因陌生而拒绝，从而错失最佳治疗时机。需要医生花费较多的时间和精力去解释。为了让患者了解这项先进有效的治疗技术，我们创作了这本通俗易懂的科普读物，作为患者了解该技术的桥梁。本书以图为主，图文并茂、通俗易懂。内容生动有趣，贴近生活。

Implant dentistry is a popular treatment with remarkable advantages. Some patients might miss the optimal opportunity of starting treatment if they are unfamiliar with the process.This pamphlet relates the treatment process to daily life and makes it easier to understand.

目录
Content

3　我能种牙吗？

4 种牙前后的有关知识

目录
Content

1 Elementary knowledge of dental implants

2 Frequently asked questions

3 Can I have an implant tooth?

4　Perioperative knowledge of implant surgery

1 种植牙基本知识

1 Elementary knowledge of dental implants

什么是种植牙？

种植牙是一种人造牙，用于替代缺失的天然牙。它有一个类似天然牙的人工牙根，能有效地行使天然牙的功能。目前的种植牙大多是由种植体（人工牙根）、基台（连接装置）和修复体（人工牙冠）三个部分组成。它的结构与功能与天然牙类似，可以完美地替代所缺失的天然牙齿，能有效地恢复美观和咀嚼功能。

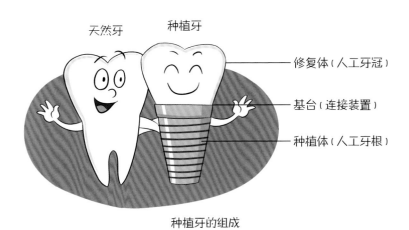

种植牙的组成

What are dental implants?

Dental implants are man-made teeth which are used to replace missing, natural teeth. They are placed on strong, artificial roots which allow the patient to chew efficiently just as with natural teeth. Modern dental implants usually consist of three parts: implants (artificial root), abutments (connection device), and prosthesis (artificial crown). Dental implants share similar structure and function to natural teeth and can restore esthetic and masticatory function.

牙齿缺失有什么危害？

前牙缺失，影响美观和发音。后牙缺失，会导致咀嚼功能的下降。缺牙时间久了，相邻的牙没有依靠会出现倾斜、移位，最终导致塞牙、龋坏，甚至牙周病。对殆的牙还会伸长，占据缺牙间隙，致使牙齿不齐。因咀嚼效率下降，还会加重胃肠负担，继而影响营养的吸收。严重者还会出现多种全身相关疾病。

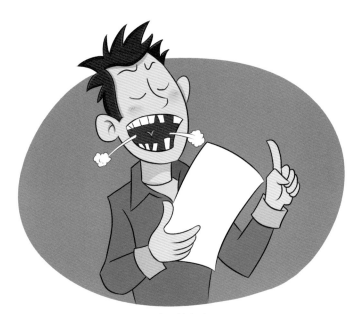

缺牙的危害

Disadvantages of missing teeth

Dentition defects or being edentulous (having no teeth) may jeopardize appearance, pronunciation, and masticatory (chewing) function. As time goes by, adjacent teeth will lean and move, resulting in food impaction, dental caries (cavities), and even periodontitis (inflammation of surrounding tissue). The nearest tooth will move to occupy the space of the missing one, and this will develop into occlusion disorder (unhealthy bite). The inefficiency of masticatory function will increase the burden on the digestive system and lower efficiency of nutrient absorption.

种牙简史

　　种牙是人类长久以来的梦想和愿望,很早就有人使用动物的牙齿、骨头和贝壳等替代缺失牙的记载。

　　历经千年,人类通过努力,终于实现了种牙的梦想,这与遨游太空一样令人振奋。

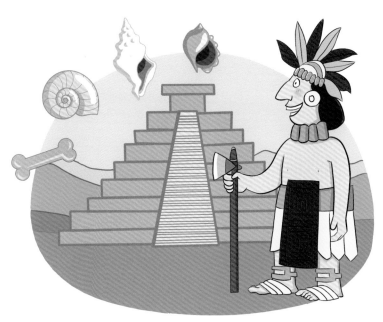

缺失牙的替代物

History of Dental Implants

Tooth replacement has been a dream of human beings since long ago. In the Inca empire, teeth were replaced with bone, shell, and animal teeth. People have been exploring different options for over one thousand years and finally made the dream come true with implant dentistry.

牙齿缺失，都有哪些修复方案？

牙齿缺失有以下三种可供选择的修复方案：

第一种：可摘义齿修复（活动义齿），将缺牙间隙两侧的牙做少许磨改，制作一个宽大的树脂义齿通过钢丝钩在相邻或者附近的牙齿上，由缺牙周围的牙、黏膜、骨组织来支持。每顿饭后必须要摘下清洗，睡前也要摘下用牙刷刷洗干净并放到有水的杯子里暂存。

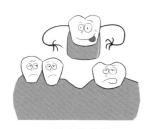

可摘义齿修复

第二种：天然牙支持式固定桥修复（固定义齿），如果缺一颗牙，必须先将缺牙间隙两侧的天然牙磨改成一定形态作为"桥墩"，再制作一副类似桥梁结构的由三个牙冠连在一起的固定桥，由医生将固定桥粘接在磨改后的"桥墩"上，从而完成修复。这种修复形式需要依靠在缺牙两侧的健康牙或牙根上，由健康牙齿或牙根来共同支持中间的缺失牙。

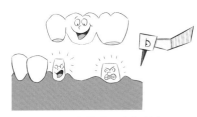

天然牙支持式固定桥修复

第三种：种植义齿修复（种植牙），如果缺一颗牙，在缺牙间隙中间直接植入一颗种植体（人工牙根）来代替缺失的天然牙根，等待几个月后，制作一个人工牙冠固定在种植上，无需依靠在缺牙两侧的任何牙齿或黏膜、骨组织上。

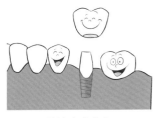

种植义齿修复

Methods of dental restoration

1. Removable partial denture

To manufacture one removable partial denture, the doctor must grind down the existing teeth near the site of the missing teeth to support the denture. The denture is mainly made of plastic and fixed to the existing teeth by steel wires. A patient with a removable partial denture should clean the denture after meals and before sleep, and store it in cool clean water.

2. Fixed bridge supported by nature teeth

To restore one missing tooth, the doctor grinds the two adjacent teeth into abutments (studs) for the bridge. A fixed bridge, which consists of three teeth, is manufactured and cemented to the studs by the dentist. The bridge is supported by the adjacent natural teeth or tooth roots.

3. Dental implant

A dental implant can be regarded as a man-made tooth root which is placed in the site of the missing tooth. After several months of healing, a crown is fixed to the implant. Neither an adjacent tooth nor gingival tissue is necessary to support the prothesis.

种植牙与其他义齿相比有哪些优点?

1. 种植牙与可摘义齿相比,不用反复摘戴,没有较大的附件,不影响发音和美观,不用依靠在邻近的天然牙和牙槽黏膜上,使用方便,寿命较长。

2. 与天然牙支持式固定桥相比,种植牙同样不需要依靠在相邻的天然牙上,因此,不用大量磨改余留的天然牙。

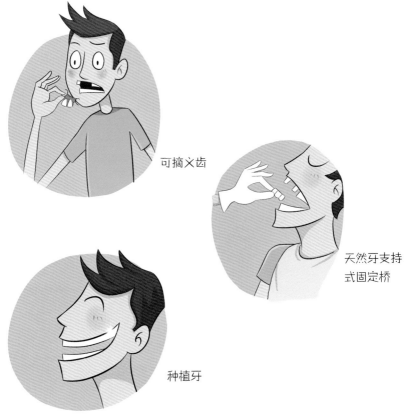

可摘义齿

天然牙支持式固定桥

种植牙

三种修复方式的对比

Advantages of dental implants over other dental protheses

1. Compared to a removable partial denture, dental implants completely avoid the trouble of removing the denture and putting it back on again. No attachments mean no interference with pronunciation and esthetics. Dental implants also last longer and cause no burden of nearby teeth and gingiva.

2. As previously mentioned, dental implants have their own roots independent of surrounding teeth. The most obvious advantage of dental implants over fixed bridges with no harm to the healthy adjacent teeth.

种植牙最大的优点是什么？

　　种植牙最大的优点在于不用依靠天然牙或黏膜来支持，不用磨改余留的天然牙。它拥有一个独立的与天然牙类似的人工牙根，因此，咬合力是通过人工牙根直接传递到颌骨中，这与天然牙的解剖生理结构类似，受力方式相同。

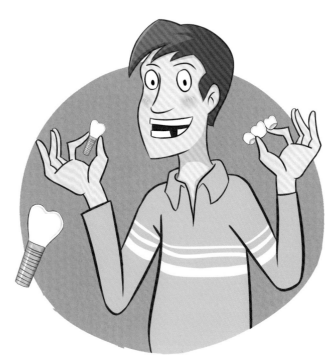

种植牙的优势

The biggest advantage of dental implants

The biggest advantage of dental implants is that they are supported by independent, artificial roots. The occlusal force is conducted to the maxilla or mandible (jaw) though the roots just as with natural teeth. No harm comes to the adjacent teeth and nearby gingiva.

种植牙有什么缺点？

相对于传统义齿修复，种植牙疗程较长，费用较高，且有一定的适应证。

目前，医学专家还在努力改良现有的医疗技术和方案，力求将疗程进一步缩短。随着新材料和新技术的不断涌现，种植牙的适应证也日益扩大。另外，激烈的市场竞争也给广大患者提供了不同品牌、不同价格产品的选择。

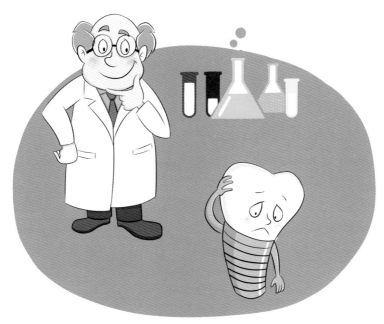

种植牙的缺点

What are the disadvantages of dental implants?

Compared with traditional dentures, dental implants have a longer duration of treatment, higher cost, and a more limited range of indications. Currently, medical experts are still improving the available technologies to shorten the course of treatment. With the emergence of new materials and technologies, the indications for dental implants are extending. Market competition provides more choices to patients in brands of implants and prices.

为什么种植牙比较贵？

种植牙是一种能长期存留在口腔中的人工装置,历经了几代人的不断探索和研究,也是各国顶尖科技人才的智慧结晶。种植牙科技含量高,工艺复杂,由多种精密配件组成,而且不少配件要个性化定制。

另外,做种植牙对医疗单位及设备要求较高,必须有现代化的诊室、手术室、口腔科 CT 机、麻醉及监护设备,以及多种特殊种植外科手术器械和口腔工艺设备等。最重要的是,还需要一个专业技术团队,其中包括有相应资质的种植外科、种植修复、牙周专科医师团队,以及受过特殊培训的医生助手、口腔技师、护理团队等多种专业技术人员。

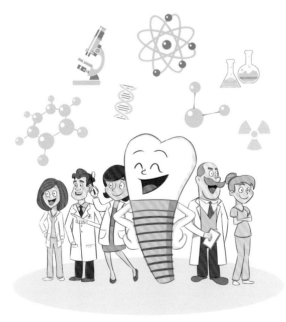

专业技术团队

Why are dental implants expensive?

Dental implants are part of a complex procedure including of custom-made components. Placing implants requires a modern consulting room, operation room, dental CT, anesthesia and monitoring equipment, as well as implant surgical instruments and oral processing equipment. Most importantly, a professional team is required, including a qualified team of implant surgeons, implant restoration specialists, periodontal specialists, as well as specially trained assistants, technicians, nursing teams, and other professional personnel.

种植牙是怎么种上去的?

种植过程基本上分为两期:

第一期:医生把人工牙根植入缺牙区,然后等 2~6 个月的时间,目的是让"人工牙根"牢牢地长在牙槽骨里。这段时间不影响您的正常工作和生活。

第二期:人工牙根长好后,您按照约定时间再回到医院或诊所,医生会在人工牙根上安装人工牙冠(也就是基台和修复体),这一步相当于量体裁衣。这时医生会根据您个人牙齿的形态、大小、颜色和排列情况来制作人工牙冠,这个牙冠的外观会与原来的缺失牙非常接近,往往可以达到以假乱真的效果。

特殊情况下也可以将两期合并,即牙根植入后即刻就连接基台并戴上人工牙冠。

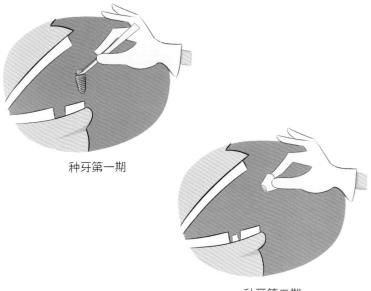

种牙第一期

种牙第二期

How is dental implantation accomplished?

The whole procedure of dental implantation consists of two steps:

1. The dentist implants an artificial root into the alveolar bone. Then, two to six months of healing is recommended. During this period of time, the patient's daily life will not be affected.

2. After healing, the dentist will manufacture a crown (abutment and prothesis) to finish the treatment. Usually, the crown is customized to fit the whole dental arch in color, size and shape. It is usually very difficult to tell a well fabricated crown from a natural tooth.

种植牙是用什么材料制作的？

　　目前种植牙的人工牙根部分是由纯钛或者钛合金制成的。表面经过特殊处理,具备良好的生物相容性,能与骨组织细胞相结合,极少会发生排异反应。牙冠部分则由全瓷、烤瓷或烤塑等材料制成。其中,全瓷冠因其优异的强度、生物相容性和美观性而得到了广泛地应用。相信在不久的将来会有更好的人工材料诞生。

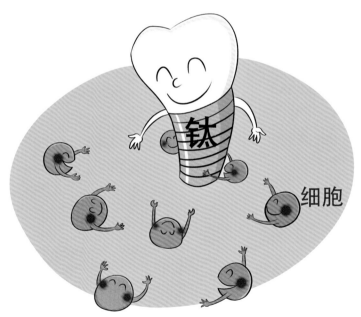

纯钛或钛合金制作的人工牙根

Materials of dental implants

The root of the dental implant is made of pure titanium or titanium alloy. The surface of the root is usually processed. The implant is so biologically friendly that osseointegration (binding implant with bone) will be complete. Rejection is rare. The crown of a dental implant is usually fabricated of all-ceramic, porcelain, or resin. Of those, the all-ceramic crown is the best in strength, esthetic, and the most biologically friendly. Maybe in near future, better materials will be invented.

人工牙根能种活吗?

人工牙根能种活。种植体(人工牙根)植入颌骨后的几个月中,周围的骨组织在种植体表面附着生长并与之牢固结合在一起,使人工牙根成为你身体的一部分,这个过程称为骨结合。这个现象是由已故的瑞典科学家 Brånemark 教授最先发现并命名的。

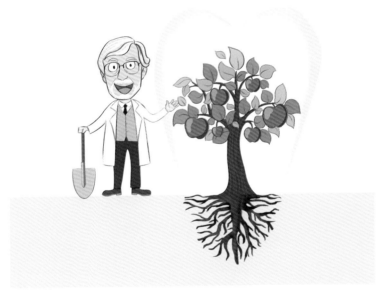

人工牙根能种活

Is the root of a dental implant alive?

Once the dental implant is inserted into alveolar bone (jaw bone), the bone tissue will grow and attach to the implant after several months of healing. This procedure makes the dental implant part of your body-'osseointegration', first named by Per-Ingvar Brånemark, a Sweden scientist.

种植牙与烤瓷牙、全瓷牙有什么不同?

烤瓷牙和全瓷牙是指制作人工牙冠的一种修复方式(例如二氧化锆全瓷牙、二硅酸锂玻璃瓷牙和烤瓷熔附金属全冠等)。在种植牙普及之前,人工牙冠多采用以上修复方式制作,并粘固在磨改后的天然牙冠上。

种植牙是指在人工牙根的基础上,选择安装以上各类人工牙冠来修复缺牙的方式。

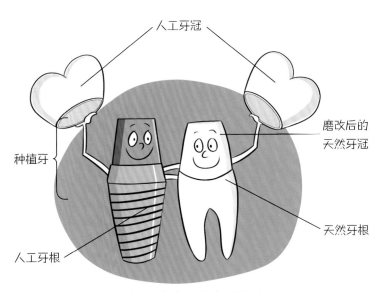

种植牙与烤瓷牙、全瓷牙的不同

What is the difference between dental implants and all-ceramic crowns or porcelain crowns?

All-ceramic crowns and porcelain crowns refer to materials and methods, such as zirconium dioxide, lithium disilicate glass, and porcelain fused to metal. Before the popularization of dental implants, the crowns were mostly made by the above materials and bonded to the natural teeth.

Dental implants refer to the method of connecting the above kinds of crowns to the artificial root to restore the missing teeth.

人工牙冠是怎么装到种植牙根上的?

人工牙冠由医生通过特殊的螺丝或者粘接方式来固位,非常牢固,患者自己不能自行取戴。只有全口牙缺失时,采用种植覆盖义齿修复的患者可以自行取戴义齿。

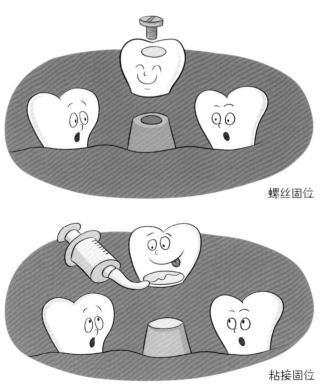

螺丝固位

粘接固位

种植牙人工牙冠的固位方式

How is the crown connected to the root of a dental implant?

Usually, the crown is connected to the root though a special screw or binding material. The connection is so strong that the patient cannot remove it. Only edentulous patients with an implant-supported overdenture can remove the denture from the implant supports.

种植牙结实吗?

正常情况下种植牙非常结实,可以承受数 10 千克以上的咬合力。

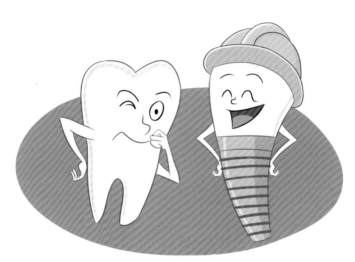

结实的种植牙

Is a dental implant strong?

A dental implant is very strong. It can withstand tens of kilograms of occlusal force.

种植牙能用一辈子吗?

若治疗顺利并维护得当,绝大多数种植牙都可以长期使用,不少种植牙甚至比天然牙齿的使用寿命还要长。

我们建议您,不论是否有种植牙,都应该每年至少进行一次口腔检查和维护,以确保牙齿的长久健康和正常使用。

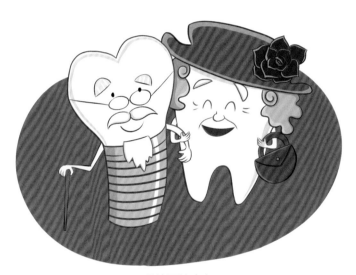

种植牙的寿命

Can a dental implant be used permanently?

If the treatment is successful and well-maintained, most people can use it permanently. Many dental implants last longer than natural teeth. We recommend all patient receive an oral examination and regular maintenance at least once per year, with or without implants.

2　我想了解的几个问题

2　Frequently asked questions

种牙痛吗?

　　种牙不会痛。种牙之前会打麻药,因此整个过程基本无任何疼痛。术后麻醉效果逐渐消散,根据手术情况和个人体质的不同,局部可能会有轻微的肿胀和不适,一般也会在 2~3 天内缓解。

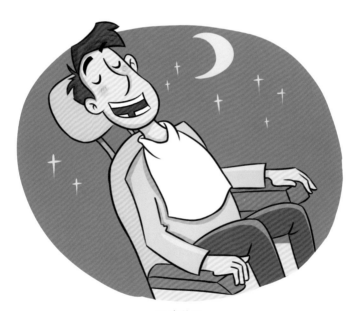

无痛种牙

035

Is placing implants painful?

Before surgery, the patient receives anesthesia that eliminates pain. After the anesthetic effect gradually dissipates, there may be slight swelling and discomfort in the local area and it is generally relieved within two to three days. The amount of discomfort varies, depending on the specific operation and differences in body mass.

种牙术后会痛吗?

　　根据手术的不同种类和创伤大小,术后 2~3 天内可能会有不适或疼痛,但一般不影响日常生活,必要时可以常规服用止疼药以缓解疼痛。

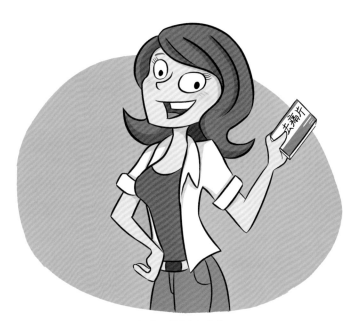

术后可服用止痛药

Is it painful after the implant surgery?

Depending on the type of surgery and the size of the wound, there may be discomfort or pain within two to three days after surgery, but it generally does not affect daily life. If necessary, you can take painkillers to relieve pain.

种牙需要多长时间？

　　植入种植体(人工牙根)是一个小手术,手术操作过程一般需要半小时,根据个人缺牙情况和手术复杂程度,有些种植手术所需时间可能会适当延长。

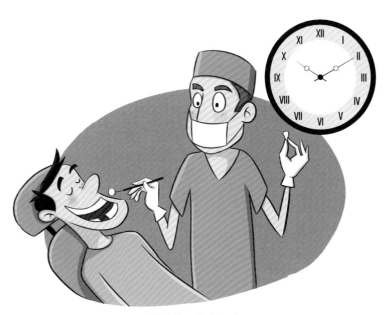

种牙是一个小·手术

How long does an implant surgery take?

Implanting an artificial root is a minor operation. The operation usually takes half an hour, but procedure time may be extended depending on the condition of individual's missing teeth and the complexity of the operation.

种植术前我还需要注意什么问题？

　　除了维护基本的全身健康状态，还应保持良好的口腔卫生状态和正常的生活作息规律，女性患者手术应该避开月经期。

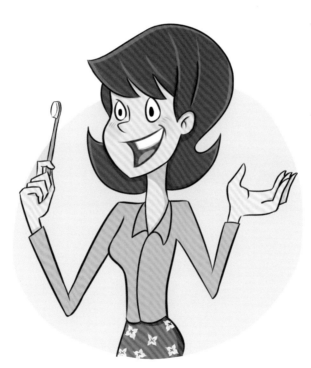

保持良好的口腔卫生状态

What else should I pay attention to before the implant surgery?

In addition to maintaining general health, it is also necessary to maintain good oral hygiene and a normal daily routine. Female patients should schedule operation on a day they are not menstruating.

种牙期间影响我的生活吗?

几乎没有影响。一般来说,种牙期间的几个月内需要复诊 3~5 次,每次都是当天内完成,不会对您的日常生活造成影响。只是在种植人工牙根手术后的 1~2 周内有一些注意事项需要遵循,例如每天口服消炎药物,吃温软饮食,避免剧烈运动等。

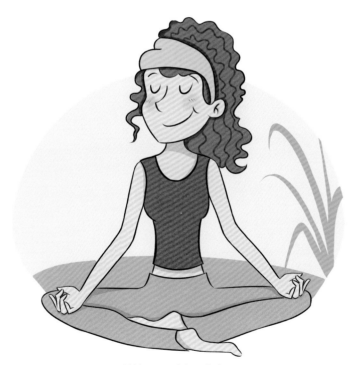

种植牙不影响日常生活

Does the dental implant healing period affect my life?

Not very much. In general, there are three to five visits within a few months of dental treatment. Each visit is expected to be completed within the same day and will not affect your daily life. During the first one to two weeks after implanting, there are some care instructions to follow: oral anti-inflammatory drugs every day, cool and soft diet, avoiding strenuous exercise, and so on.

种牙有风险吗？

　　种植牙是小型手术,一般不会对全身健康造成影响或者产生风险。与拔牙手术类似,种牙的风险取决于多种因素,多数并发症是暂时且可控制的,例如血肿、感染、出血、疼痛或其他不适等。少数情况下种植术后也可能发生局部皮肤感觉减退和麻木、软硬组织急慢性感染等情况,需要尽量防范并采取一定的治疗措施。

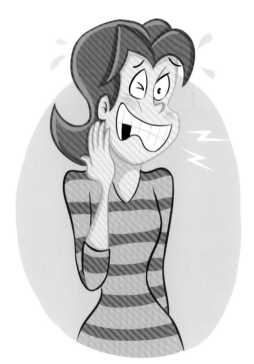

种植术后不适

Is there a risk during the dental implant procedure?

Dental implants are small operations that generally do not affect or risk the overall health. Similar to tooth extraction, the risk of dental implants depends on a variety of factors. Most complications are temporary and controllable, such as hematoma (bruise), infection, bleeding, pain, or other discomfort. In a few cases, local skin sensation decreased, numbness appeared, and acute or chronic infection of soft and hard tissue occurred after implantation.

种牙需要住院吗？

种牙不需要住院,种牙期间只需根据约定时间到医院门诊复诊几次即可,每次治疗都是在当日内完成的。

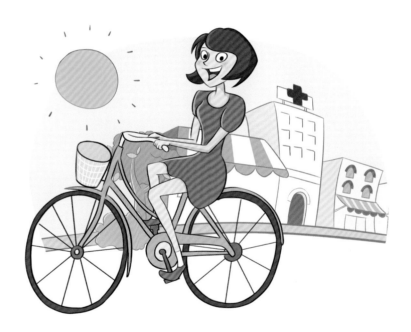

种牙无需住院

047

Is hospitalization necessary after dental implant placement?

No, each treatment is completed in one day. The patient only needs a few subsequent visits to the hospital for follow up examinations.

种植术后有哪些注意事项？

1. 术后轻咬纱布以防渗血，30~60 分钟后方可吐出，有口水可以咽下，尽量少说话。

2. 术后 2 小时方可进食，避免用手术侧咀嚼食物，宜食用稀、软、温凉的食物。

3. 术后 24 小时内请不要刷牙，以免破坏伤口凝血块，引起出血。

4. 术后几天之内，口水内含有少量血丝属正常现象，若出血较多可去医院或口腔门诊复诊。

5. 术后可根据医嘱服用抗感染、止疼药物。若 3~4 天后术区仍明显肿痛，可去医院或口腔门诊复诊。

6. 术后 7~10 天拆线。

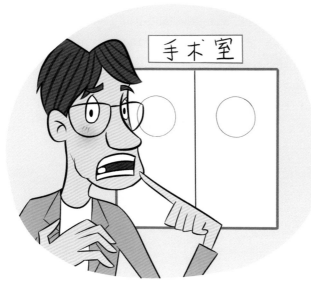

种植术后注意事项

What are the considerations after implantation?

(1) Gently bite the gauze after the operation to prevent bleeding, and spit it out after thirty to sixty minutes. Saliva can be swallowed. Speak as little as possible.

(2) Eat at least two hours after surgery, avoid chewing food on the side of surgery, and have food that is liquid, soft and cool.

(3) Do not brush your teeth within twenty-four hours after surgery, so as not to damage the blood clots in the wound and cause bleeding.

(4) Within a few days after surgery, a small amount of blood in the saliva is normal. If there is more bleeding, you can come to the hospital.

(5) Antibiotic, analgesic (anti-pain), and anti-inflammatory drugs can be taken according to the doctor's advice. If the operation area is still swollen and painful after three to four days, you can go to the hospital for a return visit.

(6) The sutures can be removed seven to ten days after surgery.

牙种好后还会出现什么问题？

虽然发生概率不高,但也可能会出现以下一些问题:

1. 种植体周围牙龈或软组织发生肿胀和溢脓,这多与口腔卫生不良有关,需要加强口腔卫生的个人维护,并定期由医生进行专业维护。

2. 种植体周围骨质发生持续性萎缩和吸收,常与口腔卫生不良、吸烟,以及糖尿病、骨质疏松症等内分泌系统疾病相关,应到医院就诊检查确定原因以便尽早治疗。

3. 由于种植体与骨组织之间没有牙周膜的缓冲,因此,基于种植体的瓷修复体发生崩瓷的概率比天然牙的瓷修复体更大一些,如果种植体没有问题,只需要重新制作人工牙冠即可。

4. 罕见情况下,可发生种植体或固位螺钉的折断,多与患者有磨牙症、咬合不平衡等问题相关,需要根据原因进行处理。

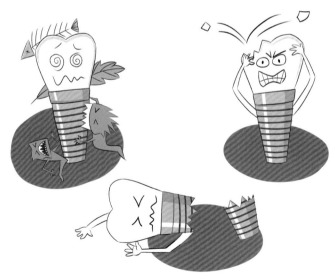

种植体可能出现的问题

What problems may happen after the end of the treatment?

Although the probability is not high, there may be some problems:

(1) The gums or soft tissue around the implant are swollen and have pus, which is related to poor oral hygiene. It is necessary to strengthen personal maintenance of oral hygiene and regular professional maintenance by doctors.

(2) Persistent wasting away and absorption of bone around the implant are related to endocrine diseases, poor oral hygiene, smoking, diabetes, and osteoporosis. The patient should go to the hospital for medical examination to determine the reason and receive treatment as soon as possible.

(3) As there is no periodontal membrane between the implant and the bone tissue, the porcelain prosthesis on the implant is more likely to experience a chip than a natural tooth. If there is no problem with the implant, the doctor will remake the crown.

(4) In rare cases, the implant or retaining screw may fracture, which is related to bruxism (grinding teeth) or an imbalanced bite.

种的牙会发炎吗?

种植牙周围的牙槽骨和黏膜也有可能发生与牙周炎类似的炎症。炎症的早期阶段只涉及黏膜而不涉及种植体周围骨组织,称为种植体周围黏膜炎,如果维护好口腔卫生并进行适当治疗,这种炎症造成的损害是可逆的。如果黏膜炎未能及时控制,则有可能伴发种植体周围牙槽骨的破坏和吸收,可称为种植体周围炎,如不及时处理则可能导致种植牙松动和失败。

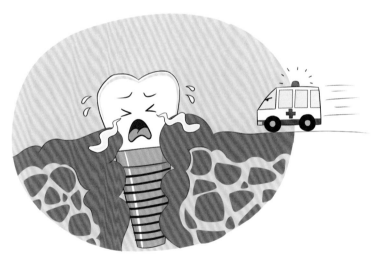

种植体周围炎

Will implants develop infection?

They can. Peri-implant mucositis may appear if oral hygiene is poorly maintained. This early stage of soft tissue inflammation can be reversed if oral hygiene is improved. Otherwise, peri-implant mucositis may progress to peri-implantitis, which involves alveolar bone loss that leads to loosening of the dental implant and implant failure.

种的牙掉了怎么办?

种植牙也可能会因为某些原因发生松动甚至脱落,例如种植体周围炎、种植体折断等,这种情况下可考虑替换一颗新的种植体或者改为其他修复形式。

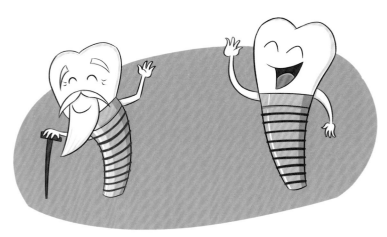

替换新的种植体

What happens if the dental implant falls off?

Dental implants may loosen or even fall off due to peri-implantitis or implant fracture. A new implant or another form of repair may be required.

别人能看出来我有种植牙吗？

精准的种植体植入与高质量的人工牙冠制作,可以确保种植牙具有天然牙的美学效果,理想的种植牙完全可以"以假乱真",您的朋友通常不会分辨出种植牙与天然牙的差别。

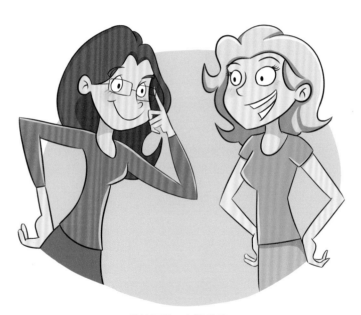

种植牙能"以假乱真"

Will others recognize my dental implant?

Precise implant placement and high-quality crown preparation ensure that dental implants have the same esthetic as natural teeth. The ideal dental implants are realistic and your friends usually cannot distinguish the difference between dental implants and natural teeth.

种植牙和天然牙一样好看吗?

"以假乱真"是牙齿修复的美学目标,种植牙由于其自身的几大优势,可以在最大程度上实现或接近这一目标。前牙美学区种植义齿修复虽然难度大,技术要求高,治疗周期长,但可以最大限度的恢复并改善您的容貌,使您重新可以轻松的开怀大笑而不必担心牙齿问题。

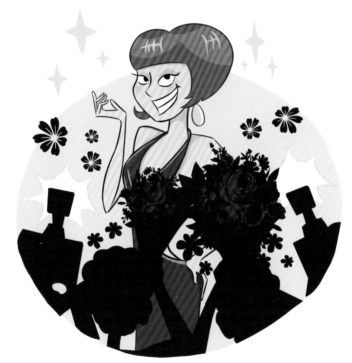

种植牙恢复容貌

Will dental implant look as good as real teeth?

Emulating natural teeth is the esthetic goal of dental restorations. Anterior implants can be difficult, with highly technical requirements and a long treatment cycle. However, once done, they can restore and improve your appearance. You will be able to laugh again without worrying about any dental embarrassment.

种植牙用起来和天然牙感觉一样吗?

种植牙几乎和天然牙一样,咀嚼时没有特别的感觉。刚戴入种植牙时会有轻微的不适和异物感,这些感觉一般会在几小时或者几天内完全消失。使用一段时间后,您不会感觉到种植牙的存在,甚至会忘记种牙的位置。

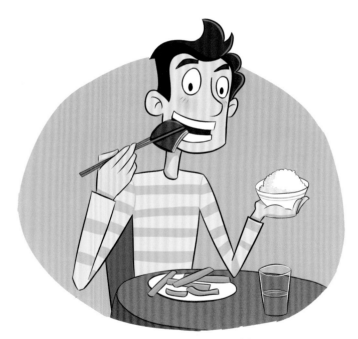

种植牙用起来和天然牙一样

Do dental implants feel like real teeth?

They feel almost the same and there is no difference when chewing. There is a slight discomfort and foreign body sensation when you wear a crown for the first time. In general, these feelings will disappear completely in hours or days. After a certain period of use, you will not feel the presence of dental implants and forget that they exist.

种植牙能咬硬物吗？

有研究表明,种植牙几乎与真牙同样稳固,能承受相当大的咀嚼力,因此咀嚼正常的饭、菜、肉等食物没有任何问题。但种植牙牙根毕竟长在牙槽骨里,骨组织承受过大的咬合力会发生应力性骨吸收,所以建议您还是要避免用种植牙咬肉干、干饼、果壳等过于坚韧的食物。

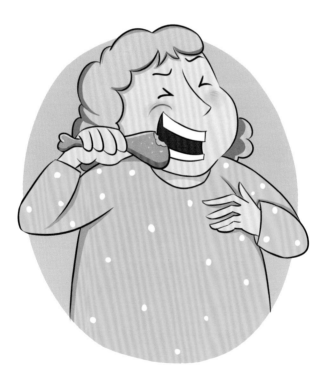

种植牙能承受正常的咀嚼力

Can I bite hard food with dental implants?

Dental implants are almost as stable as natural teeth and can withstand considerable masticatory forces. Dental implants have no problem helping patients chew foods like rice, vegetables, and meat. However, the root of the implant is in the alveolar bone and stress-induced bone resorption (bone loss) occurs when bone tissue is subjected to excessive bite force. It is recommended that you avoid using dental implants to bite jerky, dry cake, shells and other tough foods.

种完牙后能立刻咬东西吗？

种完牙后不能立刻咬东西。种植体刚植入的几周或者几个月之内，与周围骨组织的结合还不牢固，此时受力会影响种植体的愈合进程，甚至造成骨结合失败。一般建议术后两小时可食用稀、软、温凉的食物，一个月后再逐渐增加食物的硬度，直至几个月骨结合后就可以正常咀嚼了。

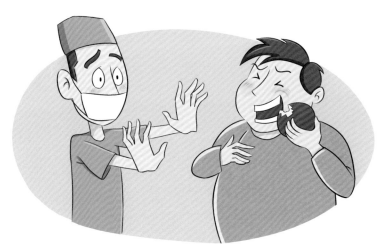

种完牙后不能立刻咬食物

Can I bite right after the surgery?

No, the process of osseointegration will not be complete until several months later. Early bite force loading will do great harm to the implant, potentially resulting in failure of osseointegration. The patient should have some cool, soft food after surgery and gradually try chewing harder food. When the osseointegration completes, months later, the patient can chew normally.

缺几颗牙就要种几颗吗？

　　并非每颗缺牙的位置都需要植入一颗种植体。植入种植体的数量，需根据您的身体情况、牙槽骨量、咬合情况以及经济承受能力等因素来综合考虑。例如，对于全口牙齿都缺失的患者，上下颌需要分别植入至少两颗种植体，便能使全口义齿获得基本的固位。如果植入四颗以上种植体，全口义齿就能像固定义齿一样不用取戴，既牢固又舒适。

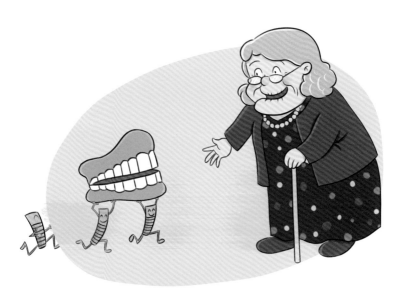

种植体辅助全口义齿固位

Does every missing tooth require an implant?

No, the number of implants depends on factors such as your physical condition, the alveolar bone mass, occlusion (bite), and economic affordability. For example, for patients missing all teeth, at least two implants will allow complete dentures to obtain basic retention. If more than four implants are placed, a complete denture can act as a fixed denture and be more stable and comfortable.

种植牙对我的余留牙有损害吗？

种植牙对余留牙不仅没有任何损害,而且还会起到保护作用。我们知道,缺牙后经常会出现邻牙的倾斜、扭转、牙间隙增大,甚至牙齿松动等一系列问题,影响咀嚼功能和面部美观。应尽早用种植牙替代缺失牙,这样就能避免继发性问题的出现,从而保护余留牙的健康。

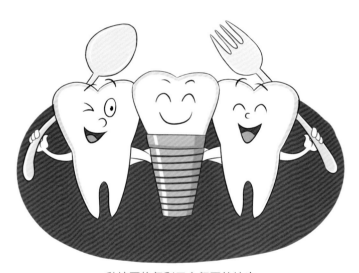

种植牙修复利于余留牙的健康

069

Does the dental implant do harm to remaining teeth?

No, to the contrary, dental implants not only avoid harming your remaining teeth, but often play a protective role. Lack of teeth often leads to inclination of the adjacent teeth, torsion (twisting) of the adjacent teeth, enlargement of diastema (tooth gap), and even loosening of the adjacent teeth (which causes a series of aggravating problems that affect masticatory function and facial appearance). Timely-placed dental implants will prevent these secondary problems and protect the remaining teeth.

牙齿拔掉能立刻种牙吗？

通常情况下，牙齿拔掉后需要等待几个月的愈合期后才可以种牙。在符合特定要求的情况下也可以即拔即种。

即拔即种又叫"即刻种植"，是指在拔牙的同时就植入种植体。即刻种植的优点是将拔牙和种牙两次手术合并成一次手术，缩短了治疗周期，减少了就诊次数，并能获得良好的美学效果。但即刻种植有一定的适应证，否则就会增加种植失败的风险，您是否适合拔牙后即刻种植最好咨询有丰富经验的医师后再作决定。

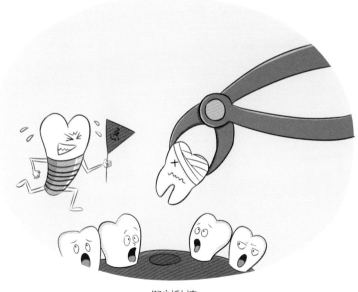

即刻种植

Can a dental implant be inserted right after tooth extraction?

Sometimes, the implantation can be done right after tooth extraction (immediate implant placement). In other cases, the tooth extraction site requires months of healing before implant placement. The advantages of immediate implant placement include reducing treatment time and better esthetic appearance. The decision to immediately place implants or to wait must be made by experienced dentists to reduce the risk of failure.

种牙期间，我不想嘴里有缺牙，能做个临时牙吗？

　　多数情况下是可以的，一般采用可摘义齿作为过渡性义齿，也可以使用固定在口内的"粘接桥"来临时修复。不论配戴哪一类临时牙，都应避免压迫到下方的种植体。

　　如果您有特殊需求，要求临时牙既美观又舒适牢固，我们也可以在刚植入的种植体上安装一个临时牙冠，称为"即刻修复"，但该方法并不能即刻恢复咀嚼功能，只能咀嚼非常软质的食物，2~6个月骨结合完成后，就可更换为永久性牙冠并正常咀嚼食物。

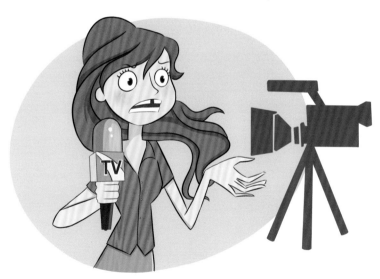

种牙期间可以做临时牙

Is a temporary denture all right during the treatment period?

Most of time, a removable partial denture or a binding bridge can be used as a temporary denture. The first issue is that neither of these temporary dentures will add stress on the implant. If the patient wants an esthetically pleasing, strong, and comfortable temporary denture, the dentist can provide a crown right after the implant surgery. This is called immediate restoration. After the immediate restoration is done, the patient is allowed to chew only very soft food. The temporary denture will finally be replaced by the permanent one after the procedure of osseointegration completes two to six months later.

为什么种牙前要拍 X 线片?

　　种植牙就像种树一样,医生要根据剩余土壤的多少来判断能不能种植或者如何种植。而且颌骨内还有不少重要的解剖结构应避免损伤。例如下颌骨中的下颌神经血管束,上颌骨内的上颌窦底黏膜。骨量、骨质以及重要解剖结构的位置和形态都需要通过拍 X 线片来确定。

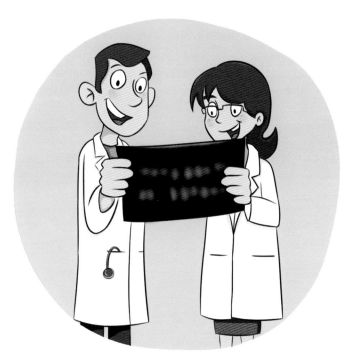

种牙前要拍 X 线片

Why is an x-ray necessary before implant surgery?

Placing a dental implant is like planting a tree. Doctors need to judge whether and how to place the implant like planting a tree according to the amount of soil. There are many important anatomical structures in the jaws that should be avoided, for example, the mandibular neurovascular bundle in the mandible and the maxillary sinus floor mucosa in the maxilla. Bone mass, bone quality and the position and shape of important anatomical structures need to be determined by the x-ray examination.

种植术前为什么要验血?

种植术前验血是为了了解患者的全身健康状况,排除严重的血液、内分泌等系统性疾病,做好针对性的术前准备。血液检查主要包括血细胞分析、出凝血功能、血液生化检查和传染病排查等内容。

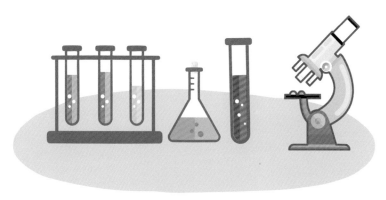

种植术前要验血

Why do I need to have a blood test before the implant surgery?

The blood test is to access the general health condition of the patient, eliminate problems from blood diseases, endocrine and other systemic diseases, and make the targeted preoperative preparation. The blood test includes blood cell analysis, blood coagulation, blood biochemistry and infectious disease.

种植牙能与天然牙一起洁牙和维护吗？

可以。与天然牙一样，对种植牙及其周围组织进行定期的洁牙和检查维护（监测）是必要的和有益的。尤其对于牙周炎的易感者和患者，其种植体周围炎的风险也较高，因此定期的口腔卫生维护和治疗尤其重要。

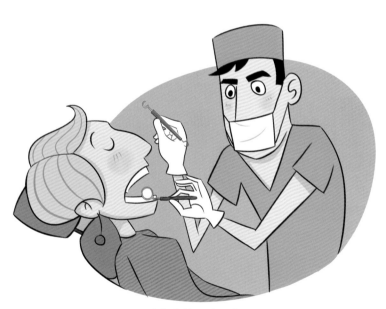

定期维护口腔卫生

079

Is the maintenance protocol of dental implant the same as natural teeth?

Yes. Periodic review of dental implant treatment is necessary and beneficial. Patients with a history of periodontitis are susceptible to an increased risk of peri-implantitis. Maintenance and periodic review with the dentist is essential.

种牙后多久复查一次？

　　口腔医生会制订一个适合您个人情况的复诊与维护计划。一般情况下，一年进行一次检查是必要的，但如果您有牙周炎病史，则建议每半年进行一次系统的检查和维护治疗。

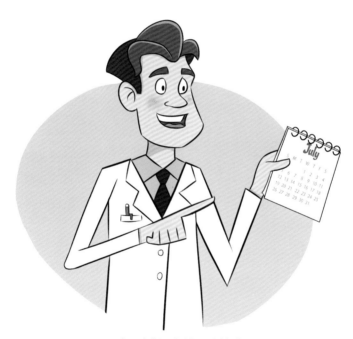

口腔医生制订复诊与维护计划

How often do I check the dental implant?

The dentist will customize a reexamination and maintenance plan that suits your personal situation. Generally, a yearly examination is necessary, but if you have a history of periodontitis, it is recommended to perform a systematic examination and maintenance treatment every six months.

种植牙如何清理维护？

种植牙的清理方法基本跟天然牙的方法一样,正确有效的刷牙就可以清理种植牙周围及其与天然牙之间的缝隙,此外,还应该定期使用牙线、牙间隙刷以及冲牙器来进行辅助性的清理。

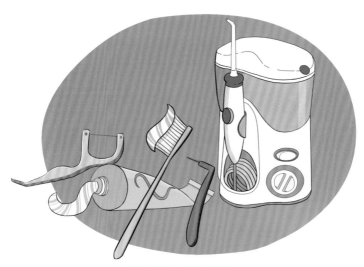

种植牙清理维护用品

How to clean and maintain the dental implant?

Cleaning a dental implant is basically the same as a natural tooth. Correct and effective brushing can clean the gap between the implant teeth and the natural teeth. Regular use of dental floss, interdental brush, and an oral irrigator should be used for additional cleaning.

3　我能种牙吗？

3　Can I have an implant tooth?

身体在什么情况下不能种牙？

　　一般来说，只有在体质非常虚弱，或者未经治疗的严重循环系统、呼吸系统及内分泌系统疾病的情况下，医生才会暂缓或者不建议进行种植牙的治疗。多数情况下，即使有心脏病、高血压、糖尿病和骨质疏松等疾病，只要得到有效的治疗和控制，也可以实施种植牙手术。

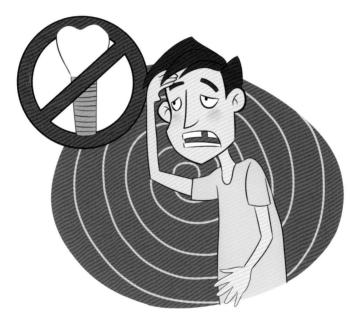

种植牙对身体条件的要求

What are the medical contraindications for implant treatment?

Patients in poor general health, with uncontrolled hematological diseases, severe respiratory diseases, or uncontrolled endocrine diseases may be restricted from dental implant surgery. Today, controlled cardiovascular diseases (e.g. heart disease, hypertension), or metabolic disorders (e.g. diabetes, hyperthyroidism), systemic bone disease (e.g. osteoporosis) are not considered absolute contraindications (impossible to receive procedure) to implant treatment. The decision should depend on medical supervision and disease management.

全口义齿易脱落,种牙能解决吗?

能解决,这正是种植牙的优势所在。如果您的牙齿掉光了,义齿没有余留牙可以固定,又不能有效的吸附在黏膜上,不仅义齿容易脱落而且还经常会有咀嚼不适或疼痛的现象,这时可以考虑选择性的植入几颗种植体,然后将义齿通过种植体固定在口内。

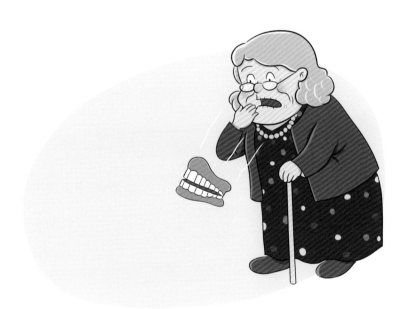

种植牙能解决全口义齿易脱落的问题

My complete denture is loose. Can dental implants solve this problem?

Yes, there is an implant application for complete denture patients. If you lost all your teeth, dentures cannot be fixed to the mucosa (soft gum tissue) effectively. This not only makes dentures fall off easily, but also often causes chewing discomfort or pain. Dental implants can be placed and the denture will be fixed to the implants in the mouth.

我的牙掉了,适合种牙吗?

这需要医生进行口腔检查和拍 X 线片后决定。一般来说,即使是老年人,只要身体健康,或慢性病患者在得到有效治疗后都可以种牙。但是青少年患者颌骨发育尚未完成,一般建议 18 岁以后再进行种植牙。

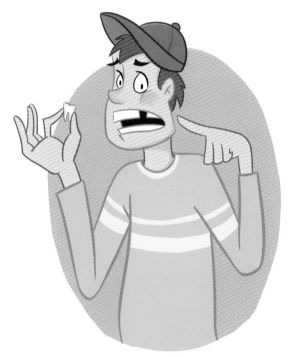

一般建议 18 岁以后再种牙

I lost my teeth. Can I have dental implants?

It depends on the oral examination and x-ray diagnosis. Even the elderly, as long as the body is healthy, or patients with chronic diseases (after effective treatment) can successfully receive dental implants. However, jaw development in adolescent patients is incomplete and dental implants are only recommended after age seventeen.

我因牙周病而缺牙，还能选择种植牙吗?

可以。不论是何种原因导致的缺牙，种植牙都是首选的治疗方案之一。

当然，您需要请医生检查后根据具体情况确定修复方案（个别情况下，若缺牙后耽误时间太久，比如几年以上就会导致牙槽骨的萎缩和丧失，会给种植修复带来困难），而且在进行种植牙之前，一般需要进行牙周基础治疗和复查控制牙周疾病，以免影响最终修复效果。

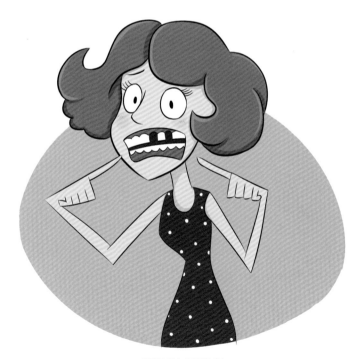

牙周病缺牙患者

I lost my teeth due to periodontal disease. Am I eligible to implant treatment?

Yes. No matter what causes the missing teeth, a dental implant is one of the first treatment options. However, the decision depends on the comprehensive examination by dental professionals. Alveolar bone atrophy (bone loss) may happen after a prolonged period of partial/complete edentulism, which may complicate the implant treatment planning. Any periodontal disease should be treated and controlled before dental implant treatment in order to avoid negative effects on the final results.

我有牙周病,可以种牙吗?

　　牙周病是发生在牙齿周围软硬组织的一类疾病,可以导致牙齿松动脱落,通常会累及区域内连续多颗牙齿,对于种植牙的牙周健康会产生不利的影响。所以,在种牙之前需要进行牙周基础性治疗,以尽可能减小牙周病对于种植牙的不利影响。牙周病患者在种牙完成后更应注意牙周健康,否则,种植牙也会发生类似牙周病的种植体周围炎。

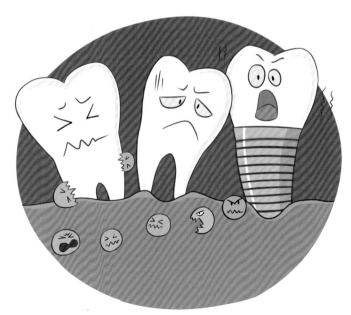

牙周病患者种牙应注意牙周健康

I have periodontitis. Am I eligible for implant treatment?

Periodontal disease is as a set of inflammatory conditions affecting the tissues surrounding the teeth, which ultimately leads to the increased mobility and/or loss of teeth. Periodontal treatment should be done before implant treatment to reduce the adverse effects of periodontal disease on implants. Patients with a history of periodontal disease are susceptible to peri-implantitis (inflammation around implant) and should be more rigorous with oral hygiene maintenance.

我正在做牙齿矫正,可以种牙吗?

原则上需要等矫正结束后才能种牙。但如果牙齿位置已经基本调整完毕,处于保持阶段,也可以提前进行种植体植入。

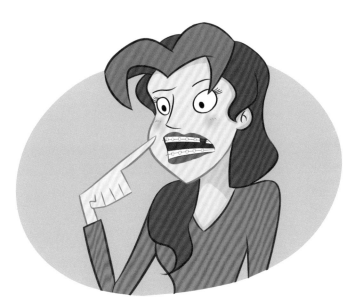

牙齿矫正的患者

I am going through orthodontic treatment. Am I eligible for implant treatment?

Implant treatment is strongly recommended after the orthodontic treatment. If the teeth movement is almost complete or is being maintained, then implants can be inserted in advance.

我是过敏体质,能种牙吗?

　　过敏体质的人可以种牙。牙种植体通常是由纯钛及钛合金制成,即使是被诊断为"过敏体质"的人,对钛发生过敏的情况也是罕见的。

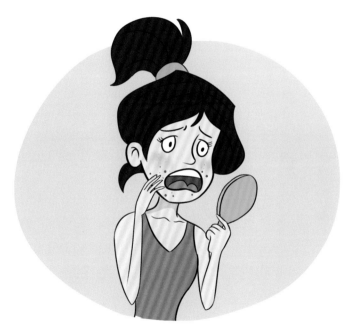

有过敏体质的患者

I have allergies. Am I eligible for dental implant treatment?

Yes. Dental implants are mostly made of pure titanium or titanium alloys, which are considered biocompatible. Few incidences of allergic reactions have been reported.

我有糖尿病,能种牙吗?

糖尿病并不是种植牙的禁忌证。但是,在开始种牙前,需要对血糖进行控制,种牙期间应特别注意避免术后感染,也可以适当延长愈合等待的时间,让种植体与骨组织结合的更牢固。

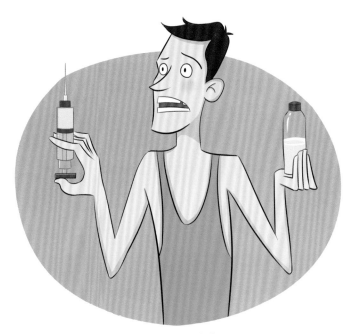

有糖尿病的患者

I am diabetic. Am I eligible for dental implant treatment?

Diabetes mellitus is not considered an absolute contraindication. However, a well-controlled blood sugar level is necessary before implant surgery. Diabetic patients are more susceptible to postoperative infection. A prolonged healing time is required to achieve better osseointegration.

我做过心脏支架（搭桥）手术，需要终生服用抗凝药物，能种牙吗？

可以种牙。对于包括种植牙在内的简单口腔手术来说，服用抗凝药物并非禁忌证。建议您将抗凝药的使用情况告知医生。

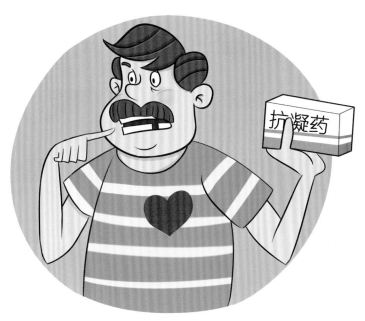

服用抗凝药物的患者

103

I have a heart bypass and am taking an anticoagulant (blood thinner). Am I eligible for dental implant treatment?

Yes. In most cases, taking an anticoagulant is not a contraindication to simple oral surgery, including dental implant surgery. We recommend that you inform your doctor of the oral anticoagulant therapy.

我曾因为高血压和心脏病住过医院,可以种牙吗?

只有极少数较为严重的心血管疾病患者不适宜种牙。例如,心肌梗死发作的 6 个月之内不宜进行种植手术;频繁发生心绞痛期间不宜进行种植手术。对于此类严重的心血管疾病患者,最好在咨询并获得专科医师的建议后再进行种植治疗。

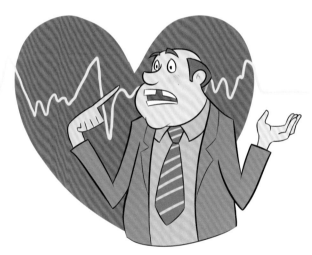

有心血管疾病的患者

I was once hospitalized for hypertension and heart disease. Am I eligible for dental implant treatment?

Absolute cardiovascular contraindications to dental implant treatments are rare, except for a few serious cardiovascular diseases. However, a recent heart attack in the past six months and unstable angina are absolute contraindications for implant surgery. For patients with severe cardiovascular disease, it is best to consult with a specialist before getting a dental implant.

怀孕期和哺乳期能种牙吗?

尽管种植牙属于简单手术,但怀孕期间最好避免进行种植。因为术后可能服用的抗生素或抗炎药物会增加胎儿生长发育方面的风险。

哺乳期内可以种牙。在因治疗需求而服用抗生素或抗炎药物的期间,我们建议可以暂停哺乳几天。

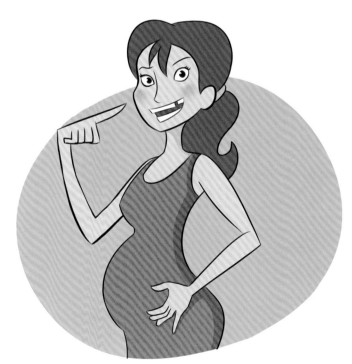

孕期避免种牙

107

I am pregnant/breastfeeding. Am I eligible for dental implant treatment?

Deferring implant surgery during pregnancy is strongly recommended. Patients may be prescribed antibiotics after implant surgery, which may increases the risk of abnormal fetal growth and development. Implant surgery during lactation is safe. However, a temporary interruption of breastfeeding is usually suggested during the period of taking antibiotics or anti-inflammatory drugs for treatment needs.

我患有较为严重的骨质疏松症,可以种牙吗?

骨质疏松并不是种植牙的禁忌证。有科学研究表明,患有和未患有骨质疏松症患者的种植成功率和存留率并没有明显的区别。然而,在考虑是否进行种植牙手术时,长期服用二膦酸盐药物的患者有发生骨坏死的风险,这需要引起注意。

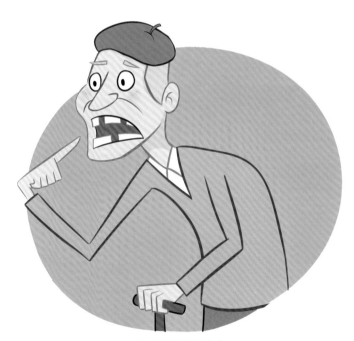

有骨质疏松的患者

109

I have severe osteoporosis. Am I eligible for dental implant treatment?

Osteoporosis is not considered as an absolute contraindication to implant treatment. There is some evidence suggesting no significant difference in implant success rate and survival rate between patients with and without osteoporosis. However, it should be noted that patients under bisphosphonate therapy are prone to develop medication-related osteonecrosis (bone tissue death) of the jaw and should be carefully assessed by dental professionals before implant surgery.

我已经 70 多岁了,还能种牙吗?

高龄并非种植禁忌证,对于 70 岁甚至是 80 岁以上的老年人,只要做好术前准备,掌握适应证,也完全可以获得理想的种植修复效果。

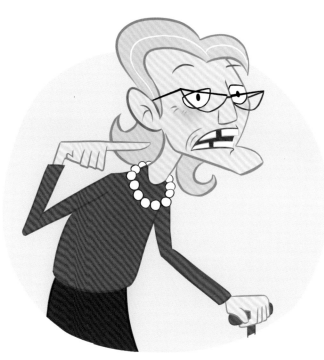

高龄老人

I am in my 70s. Am I eligible for implant treatment?

Advanced age is not a contraindication to implant treatment. With regard to higher aged patients (70+ years old), a good result of dental implant treatment could be achieved through high quality clinical management.

我不到 18 周岁，可以种牙吗？

　　种植牙是一种永久性的固定修复体，应该等到青春期结束后再进行。否则可能会干扰骨骼和牙齿正常的生长发育。对于未满 18 周岁的青少年，也可以先咨询医生，选择一些过渡性的修复方案解决美观和功能问题。

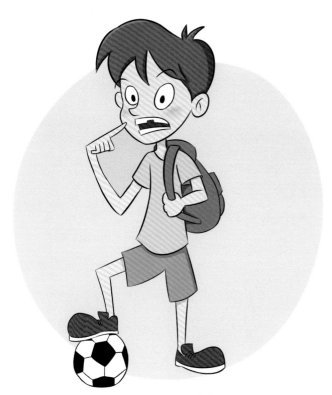

未满 18 周岁的患者

I am under 18 years old. Am I eligible for implant treatment?

Implant treatment is a permanent fixed restoration and is recommended only for patients eighteen years old or older, because there is continued skeletal growth and dentoalveolar (teeth and jaw) change during adolescence. Patients under eighteen requiring dental implant treatment should receive provisional options to restore aesthetics and function until bone development stops.

4 种牙前后的有关知识

4 Perioperative knowledge of implant surgery

种植牙对我的发音唱歌有影响吗?

不影响发音或者唱歌。种植牙能完美恢复缺失牙的形态,也没有其他阻碍发音的部件,无异物感,美观舒适,不影响发音或者唱歌。

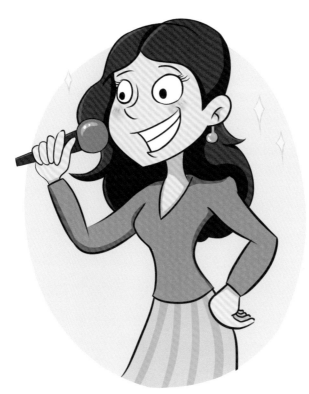

种植牙不影响唱歌

117

Will a dental implant affect my pronunciation in singing?

No, dental implants can restore the shape of missing teeth without any other component that could become an obstacle to pronunciation. Dental implants cause no sensation of something in the mouth, and they look esthetically pleasing, comfortable, and will not affect pronunciation or singing.

种牙前需要戒烟吗?

　　种牙前最好戒烟,虽然也有不少患者在吸烟的状态下顺利完成了种植牙修复,但吸烟对种植体的骨结合有确定性的负面影响,也会增加种植修复完成后种植体周围炎的发生率。因此,为了降低种植失败的概率,减少骨吸收,我们强烈建议吸烟者在种植治疗开始之前一定要戒烟。

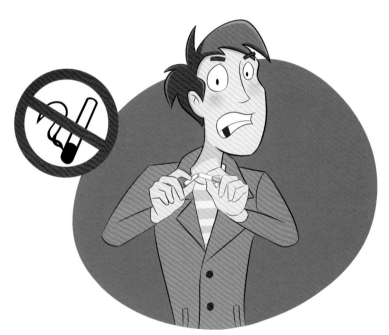

种牙前需戒烟

Do I need to quit smoking before implant treatment?

Smokers are strongly encouraged to quit smoking before implant treatment in order to reduce the risk of implant failure. There is increased risk of implant failure and peri-implantitis in smokers when compared to non-smokers.

我被告知术中需要"植骨",种牙为什么要植骨?

如同天然牙根一样,种植牙根也需要置于健康牢固的骨组织中,才能长久稳定的发挥咀嚼功能。如果您的牙槽骨不够厚实,可能会导致种进去的人工牙根不牢固,容易失败,就像大树需要有足够厚度的坚实土壤来支撑一样。因此,如果因为各种原因导致您的牙槽骨量不足,医生将通过植入人工骨粉或者自体植骨的方法来增加骨量,统称为植骨。

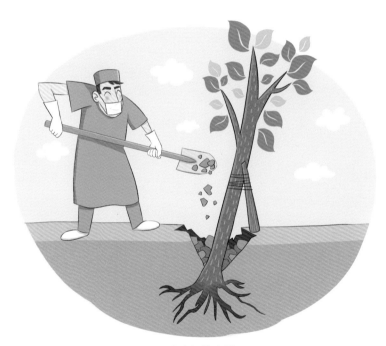

比喻植骨的必要

121

I was told that there was a need for "bone grafting" during the surgery. Why?

Just like natural tooth roots, the implants need to be placed in healthy, solid bone tissue for long-term, stable chewing. If your alveolar bone is not dense enough, it may cause the implant to become prone to failure, just as large trees need to be supported by solid soil. If your alveolar bone volume is insufficient, the doctor will place artificial bone powder or an autogenous bone graft (from your body).

医生告诉我要进行"上颌窦底提升术",为什么要这样做?

　　上颌骨内有左右两个气化的空腔,被称为上颌窦,与鼻腔是相通的。当上颌窦体积过大,牙槽骨组织过少过薄时,上颌的这个缺牙区域就没有足够的骨量来植入种植体,此时医生就要"填湖造地",即在黏膜与骨壁之间植骨以增加骨量,形成的新骨使植入的种植体更加牢固。

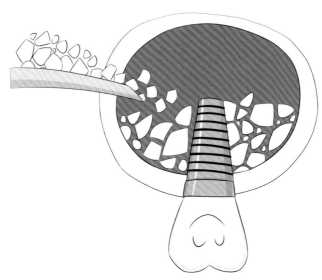

上颌窦底提升是为了加固种植体

The doctor told me to carry out "Maxillary Sinus Floor Elevation." Why?

There are two gasified cavities in the maxilla, known as the maxillary sinuses, which connect to the nasal cavity. When the maxillary sinus is too large and the alveolar bone tissue is too thin, there will not be enough bone for the dental implant. At this time, the doctor will graft bone between the mucous membrane and the bone wall to increase the bone mass, and the new bone formed will provide the necessary conditions for the dental implant.

种植牙会影响磁共振或者 CT 检查吗?

种植牙不会影响磁共振或者 CT 检查。传统义齿中含有大量普通金属,例如钴铬或者镍铬合金等,这些类型的金属会在磁共振和 CT 的图像中产生大范围的伪影和干扰,影响诊断的准确性。种植牙的体积很小,而且钛金属本身就不易产生伪影,其上部的全瓷冠更不会产生伪影。因此,种植牙基本不会影响以后做磁共振和 CT 检查。

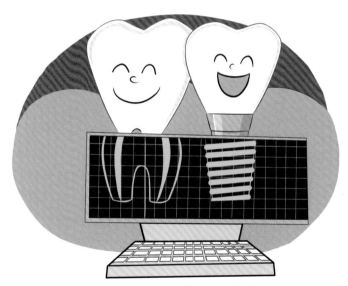

植牙不会影响磁共振和 CT 检查

Do dental implants affect MRI or CT examination?

No. Traditional dentures contain metals such as cobalt-chromium or nickel chromium alloys. These metals can produce artifacts (unwanted shapes that appear in MRI and CT images), affecting the accuracy of diagnosis. Dental implants are small in size. Titanium and ceramic crowns produce less-visible artifacts and do not negatively affect MRI or CT scans.